The Ultimate Paleo Diet Guide for Beginners and Diabetics Learn The Secrets of The Caveman Diet

by Carolyn C. Smith

1

Income Disclaimer

This book contains business strategies, marketing methods and other business advice that, regardless of my own results and experience, may not produce the same results (or any results) for you. I make absolutely no guarantee, expressed or implied, that by following the advice below you will make any money or improve current profits, as there are several factors and variables that come into play regarding any given business.

Primarily, results will depend on the nature of the product or business model, the conditions of the marketplace, the experience of the individual, and situations and elements that are beyond your control.

As with any business endeavor, you assume all risk related to investment and money based on your own discretion and at your own potential expense.

Liability Disclaimer

By reading this book, you assume all risks associated with using the advice given below, with a full understanding that you, solely, are responsible for anything that may occur as a result of putting this information into action in any way, and regardless of your interpretation of the advice.

You further agree that our company cannot be held responsible in any way for the success or failure of your business as a result of the information presented in this book. It is your responsibility to conduct your own due diligence regarding the safe and successful operation of your business if you intend to apply any of our information in any way to your business operations.

Terms of Use

You are given a non-transferable, "personal use" license to this book. You cannot distribute it or share it with other individuals.

Also, there are no resale rights or private label rights granted when purchasing this book. In other words, it's for your own personal use only.

Contents

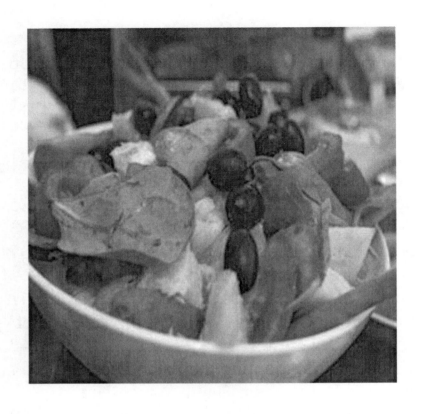

The Pros and Cons of the Paleo Diet

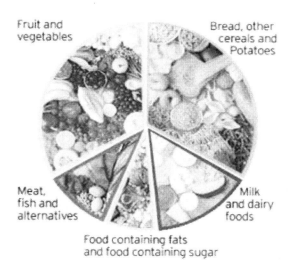

Fruit and vegetables

Bread, other cereals and Potatoes

Meat, fish and alternatives

Milk and dairy foods

Food containing fats and food containing sugar

The paleo diet is an awesome diet that has thousands of fans all over the world. People have lost weight, reduced allergies, gained control of their health issues like diabetes, cholesterol, etc. and much more with the paleo diet. In fact, it is considered one of the best diets around.

However, no diet is perfect and the paleo diet is no different. It has its pros and cons which this book will discuss. You will have to decide for yourself if the pros outweigh the cons. Thousands of people decided that it did and adopted this diet.

First, you will need to understand the paleo diet. It is a diet that is more concerned with food choices rather than calories, nutrient timing, carb cycling, detoxing, etc. In theory, the paleo diet is simple. Eat these foods and avoid these other foods. All you need to do is follow the food list. In practice, however, the paleo diet is extremely difficult in the beginning because it involves sacrifice. Nobody likes that. You are encouraged to eat grass-fed meats such as beef, poultry, bison, turkey, pork, etc.

Fish is good too. Especially wild salmon that is rich in omega-3 fatty oils. You may consume fruit and non-starchy vegetables such as broccoli, carrots, cabbage, cauliflower, green beans, spinach, etc. You may consume nuts such as pecans, almonds, walnuts and cashews. Peanuts are NOT allowed.

Eggs and plant based oils are also encouraged. Coconut oil, olive oil, macadamia oil, etc. are sources of fat. These foods are an integral part of the paleo diet.

The foods that are not allowed are grains, such as oats, wheat, barley, and rice. You're also not allowed to consume starchy vegetables, such as potatoes and corn. All dairy products are not allowed. Sugar, processed meats such as hot dogs, salami, etc. are a big no-no. Salty food, processed foods, refined foods are all not allowed.

This eliminates a huge chunk of foods that people are normally used to eating. This is one of the biggest pros of the paleo diet. Most of the foods not allowed are unhealthy and some foods such as soya beans and grains just do not go down well with most people.

The paleo diet is rich in protein and it keeps your blood sugar levels stable and prevents insulin spikes. This prevents weight gain. The diet is also very clean and that means it is anti-inflammatory. Most people on normal diets often complain of aches and pains for no reason.

This is due to cell inflammation from food that is not good. No such problems with the paleo diet. These are some of the pros of the paleo diet.

There are a few cons. This diet is not suitable for vegetarians. Paleo dieters often do not balance their meals well. Too much protein is consumed without adequate carbs. So, they'll need to carefully keep track of what they eat. When food choices are limited, more attention is required to keep the diet balanced. The paleo diet can seem too rigid and strict to many people. So, many drop off the diet.

You will need to assess your goals and weigh your options. If you're willing to make sacrifices for better health and fewer health issues, you definitely want to adopt the paleo diet. It is well worth the effort.

What Is The Paleo Diet

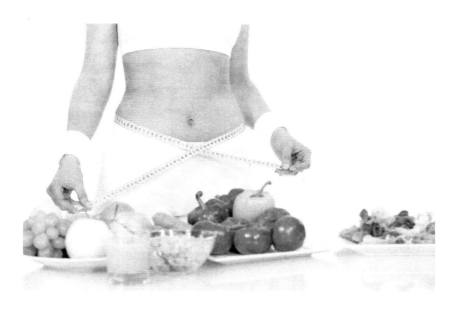

The paleo diet, also popularly known as the 'caveman' diet is a dietary plan roughly based on what our ancestors consumed during the paleolithic era. The current day diet is not an exact replication of their diet. Just a concept of what their diet would have been like – basically healthy, wholesome food that is not full of additives, preservatives and other harmful substances so often found in our current diet.

The paleo diet has seen a surge in popularity with thousands of people extolling its benefits. Books on the subject such as The Paleo Solution by Robb Wolf have becoming bestsellers. There is no denying that the paleo solution works and it is a healthy way of life. The diet itself is simple. There is a list of foods you can eat and a list of foods that you can't eat. The simplicity stops there. The difficulty arises when one has to strictly adhere to the foods that you can eat.

Most of us grew up on cereal, bread, milk, chocolates, burgers, ice-creams, etc. Foods that we have grown to love. In fact, we love these foods so much that obesity has reached epidemic proportions.

While most normal diets give you a list of foods that are not good for you, the paleo diet goes one step higher and just strikes off ingredients. For example, a normal diet will state that you should not eat doughnuts. The paleo diet states that you will not consume sugar. With this one condition, it has just eliminated a huge chunk of foods. Grains are also not allowed. Really? Yup. That means that bread, pizzas, burgers, etc. are out too. So, are processed meats such as hot dogs, salami, etc. You are only expected to eat grass fed meats, fish, poultry, fruit, non-starchy vegetables such as broccoli, cauliflower, carrots, lettuce, spinach, etc. Eggs and vegetable oils such as olive oil, coconut oil, macadamia oil, etc. are allowed as fats. You can only consume these foods.

There are a few other foods you can consume while on the paleo diet. It would be best to get a paleo cookbook and learn what you can eat and how to transform these foods into tasty dishes. Paleo dishes can be tasty too. Just because the diet is restrictive does not mean that it has to be boring. In fact, it is highly advisable that you have as many paleo recipes as possible at your fingertips. Since you have sacrificed so many foods that you considered delicious, your body will be craving these forbidden foods. Tasty paleo dishes will ease the mental torture.

Once you have gotten used to the diet, naturally your cravings will slowly decrease till there are none left. In fact, even the smell of junk food may turn you off in the future. Your body will be used to healthy food and will be repulsed by food that is not good for it.

You will be leaner, healthier and feel much better. These are the priceless benefits of the paleo diet and worth all the sacrifice. It would be great to incorporate an exercise program into your daily schedule so that you reap the full benefits of a healthy lifestyle. Then, you will truly be fit and fabulous.

PALEO ZONE SHOPPING LIST

chefkatelyn.com

Produce:

- SPINACH
- ROMAINE
- MIXED GREENS
- AVOCADO
- TOMATOES
- ONIONS

- CARROTS
- CUCUMBERS
- CELERY
- KALE
- BERRIES
- MUSHROOMS

- BELL PEPPERS
- APPLES
- BROCCOLI
- BRUSSELS SPROUTS
- ZUCCHINI
- LEMONS + LIMES

Meat:

- CAGE FREE, ORGANIC EGGS
- ORGANIC BACON
- CHICKEN BREAST, THIGHS, GROUND
- PORK LOIN, CHOPS, SHOULDER
- LAMB SHOULDER, CHOPS, GROUND
- BEEF SIRLOIN, STEAK, PRIME RIB, GROUND

Pantry:

- OILS (PUMPKIN SEED, AVOCADO, OLIVE, COCONUT)
- CANNED + PACKAGED TUNA
- ALMOND + SUNFLOWER SEED BUTTER
- BALSAMIC VINEGAR
- ORGANIC ESPRESSO BEANS
- RAW HONEY + LOCAL MAPLE SYRUP
- SEA SALT

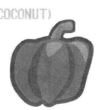

#FITFLUENTIAL

The Ultimate Paleo Guide

Recommends that you visit:

www.eatinghealthytoloseweight.net

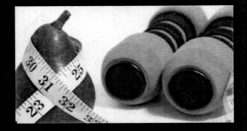

Will the Paleo Diet Help With Diabetes

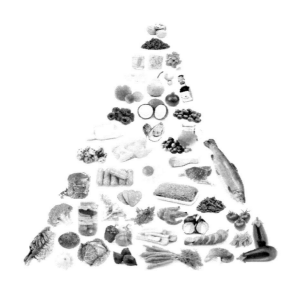

The paleo diet is one of the best ways of combating diabetes and keeping it under control. There is absolutely no doubt about this. Thousands of people who were suffering from diabetes reported benefits after adopting the paleo diet.

The paleo diet focuses mostly on eating meat, healthy fats and whole vegetables that are beneficial to the body. Sugars, simple carbohydrates, refined foods, potatoes, etc. are not allowed in the paleo diet. By following the paleo diet assiduously, one will keep their blood sugar level stable and there will hardly be any insulin spikes.

This is one of the major benefits of the paleo diet and it is exactly why the diet is so suitable for diabetes sufferers.

The key to keeping diabetes and its ill effects under control is by keeping your blood sugar stable. That is the cornerstone to staying healthy despite having diabetes. The normal way to keep diabetes under control will be to use medication, which is what most doctors will prescribe.

However, many patients have still reported having diabetic ulcers, unexplained fluctuations in blood glucose levels and other issues. The reason for this is that the foods they are consuming are not suitable for diabetic patients. The paleo diet eliminates most of these 'problem' foods.

Another problem that many diabetics face is cravings for sweet foods or foods that are not

ideal for them. These cravings are often caused by poor food choices. The more sugary foods you consume, the greater your cravings for sugary foods will be. It's a vicious cycle.
The paleo diet puts an end to all these cravings since it eliminates sugar from the diet. It may be difficult in the beginning to adapt this diet, but once you have adapted and accepted it, your cravings will disappear and your life will become much easier. You will not face a mental struggle and guilty feelings by fighting or giving in to cravings.

When blood sugar levels spiral out of control, insulin is often required to stabilize the blood sugar levels. Often, these require professional medical treatments that are time consuming and expensive. The simple fact is that it is relatively easy to keep blood sugar levels under control. Not only will you be spared the hassle of making and keeping medical appointments, but you'll also save money.

Eating foods that have a high glycemic index will send your blood sugar levels through the roofs. An example of a high GI food would be a bowl of sugary cereal. A much wiser choice would be 2 half boiled eggs with a light dash of pepper.

What's the difference?

The doughnuts are not allowed if you're on the paleo diet. The eggs are allowed and recommended. The former will give you health problems while the latter will be beneficial for your well-being. Since the paleo diet will also result in you shedding the excess pounds, you will also end up leaner and healthier. It's a win-win situation. If you're a diabetic, you definitely want to look into the paleo diet and give it a try. It might change your life for the better.

Is it Difficult to Adopt a Paleo Diet Lifestyle?

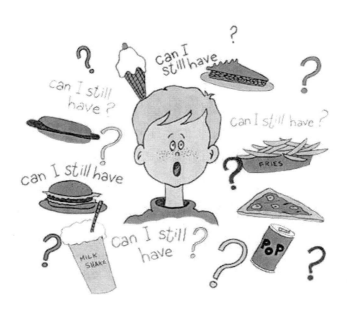

This is a difficult question to answer because it's all relative. What may seem easy to one person may be difficult to answer. That being said, the paleo diet is slightly more difficult to follow than other diets. Don't let that discourage you though. The paleo diet is also more effective than most other diets.

The paleo diet aims to remove unhealthy and even toxic foods from our diet. It is not about calories, carb consumption or other normal factors that most diets concern themselves with. The paleo diet is about eating food in its natural form without additives, preservatives and other substances that most people can't even pronounce.

Grains, sugar and certain other foods are not allowed. These foods are not suitable for human beings. Our early ancestors did not consume these foods and since the paleo diet resembles a caveman's diet, we are not supposed to eat these foods too.

This makes it difficult for many people who have lived all their lives eating foods that contain ingredients not allowed in a paleo diet. The exclusion of grain means that all breads and pastries are now not allowed. Not eating sugar means giving up comfort foods such as cookies, cakes, ice-cream, etc. It's all just overwhelming.

The question then arises… What can we eat?

Even salt is severely limited. Meats such as sausages, salami, etc. are not allowed. This can seem almost depressing. The paleo diet also encourages people to cook their own food since most of the commercially available foods do not meet paleo standards.

This is another hassle. Grocery shopping and cooking. Furthermore, paleo dieters cook their food in big batches to last a few days. All this definitely takes effort. The diet also recommends eating organic produce and grass-fed meats. This can be expensive and that is another factor that can demoralize a new paleo dieter. However, one need not be so rigid and eat only organic produce or grass-fed meats. Normal meat and veggies will do if your budget is not big.

Despite all these conditions and sacrifices, thousands of people all over the world give glowing testimonials and reviews of the paleo diet. It has made people lose weight, feel ache and pain free, lower diabetes symptoms and effects, have a healthier relationship with food, have less allergies and much more.

The sacrifices you make in the beginning will bring you rewards in the future. Once you conquer your sugar cravings, after 2 or 3 months, you will not have them anymore. A body that is getting all the nutrients it needs does not get cravings. In fact, if you will just try out the paleo diet for 3 weeks or a month, you will automatically see and feel the difference.

This is intangible and must be experienced to understand the benefits of a paleo diet.
If you have the determination and are willing to go through the 'hard yards' in the beginning, you will become healthy, happy and proud of your achievements later on. Mastering the paleo lifestyle is indeed an achievement. It takes effort and dedication just like all the best things in life. The paleo diet is one of them.

The Paleo Diet or Low Carb Diet? Which is better?

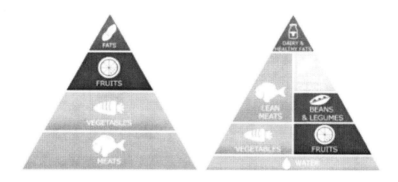

This is an excellent question and a very popular one too. It is often asked by people who are trying to lose weight and are trying to make sense of all the weight loss information floating around. This question is not really an easy one to answer because it all depends on the person adopting the diet.

This article will state the pros and cons of each diet and in the end, the decision lies in the hands of the reader. One diet is slightly better than the other but it's more difficult to adopt. So, decide wisely.

The paleo diet is not really about weight loss. It is more concerned with healthy food choices. Eating food that is good for your body and avoiding food that is not. The paleo diet is highly effective and as a result, people lose weight and this creates the idea that the paleo diet is about weight loss.

You will be eating lots of meat while on the paleo diet. Grass fed meats, eggs, healthy fats such as coconut oils and grass fed butter, etc. You will not be allowed to eat anything containing sugar, grains and refined or processed products.

This is extremely difficult for many people because they will have to give up many of their favorite foods. It's a huge sacrifice for them. This makes the paleo diet much more difficult to adopt than the low carb diet. However, if you conquer your cravings and adopt the paleo diet, you will lose weight, look better and be healthier.

You will have fewer allergies, fewer potential health issues and a better relationship with food. The cravings will disappear in about 2 to 3 months. Your weight loss will be permanent and you will have a much lower chance of gaining weight since your blood sugar levels will be stable and there will not be any insulin spikes from high GI foods.

The low carb diet on the other hand, advocates a diet that is extremely low in carbs or even in some cases, no carbs are allowed. Unlike the paleo diet which recommends a certain amount of carbs from vegetables and fruit.

A low carb diet may mean that you can consume carbs but in small quantities. Many dieters make the mistake of consuming carbs such as whole wheat bread or 'healthy' cereals. Even small amounts of these carbs will cause insulin spikes.

A low carb diet also leaves people feeling lethargic and irritable. The human body needs a certain amount of carbohydrates. If you consume too little, your metabolic rate will drop. Unlike the paleo diet which encourages the consumption of nutrient dense foods, which may make up for the lack of carbs, the low carb diet does not do that.

All too often, the dieters on the low carb diet consume too few calories and this impedes their fat loss progress. The only positive thing about the low carb diet is that it has much more leeway in its food choices. It's not as harsh as the paleo diet. No foods are forbidden in a low carb diet.

There may even be cheat days which allow you to gorge yourself and leave you lying somnolent on a couch unable to move. The paleo diet has no cheat days.
To summarize, if you have the discipline and determination, go for the paleo diet and you will have a diet that will last you a lifetime. Your health will improve vastly and you'll feel great.

If you just can't muster the determination to avoid your favorite foods, then go for the low carb diet. But, do remember that this is a short term solution. You will always be in a battle to fight the bulge. The cause of weight gain is poor food choices. So, no poor food is better than low quantities of poor food. In the end, it's your choice.

Is the Paleo Diet As Healthy As It Claims To Be?

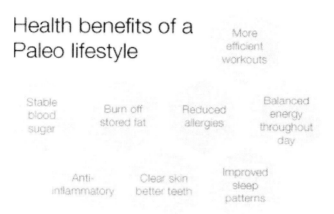

Health benefits of a Paleo lifestyle

More efficient workouts

Stable blood sugar

Burn off stored fat

Reduced allergies

Balanced energy throughout day

Anti-inflammatory

Clear skin better teeth

Improved sleep patterns

In one word…Yes. It really is.

We live in a world that is surrounded by hype, slick marketing, misleading ads, fads, crazes and short term fixes. It is easy and even understandable if you feel that the paleo diet could be all hype. Like the saying goes, all foam and no beer.

However, you will be mistaken. The paleo diet is everything it claims to be. It will improve your health, leave you looking leaner and fitter and will change your life. The paleo diet recommends only eating wholesome foods and avoiding foods that are not good for you.

For example, the paleo diet recommends eating wild caught salmon which are rich in omega-3 fatty acids. This is extremely beneficial. The current American diet is short on omega-3 acids and high in omega-6 acids. You want balance. The omega-3 acids have anti-inflammatory properties. Thousands of people suffer from inflammation due to the consumption of food that does not agree with them. The end result is aches and pains all over the body.

The paleo diet does not allow the consumption of sugar and grains. This eliminates a huge number of foods that most people are used to. Cereals, breads, pasta, pizza, cakes, chocolates, etc. By eliminating these foods, your blood sugar levels will be stable. This is excellent.

Why?

When your blood sugar levels spike, your body releases insulin. Over time the body loses insulin sensitivity and this results in increased fat storage. The moment you consume a bowl of sugary cereal in the morning, your blood sugar will shoot up and insulin will be released. Later on, you will have a sugar crash and end up feeling lethargic. Why do you think people often feel sleepy after a heavy lunch? This is the reason.

The paleo diet will keep your blood sugar levels stable. Because of this, you will not gain weight easily. Furthermore, by eliminating a huge chunk of unhealthy carbs, you will also lose all the excess weight you're carrying (provided you are on a calorie deficit) while you are on the paleo diet. People suffering from diabetes have often seen relief from the paleo diet. It is much easier to keep a steady blood glucose level while on a paleo diet.

The diet involves consuming a fair amount of meat. This ensures that you have sufficient protein for muscle building and repair. It would be wise to balance your diet with vegetables. One mistake many paleo dieters make is that they neglect to balance their meals. So, they often end up eating too much protein and not enough carbohydrates. The macronutrients must be well balanced. The correct proportion of fats, carbs and protein.

You should grab a book on paleo eating and lifestyle to learn more. There are many more pointers and tips that are beyond the scope of this article. The most important point to take away from this article is that paleo dieting is indeed healthy and sustainable over the long run. You can stay on it for the rest of your life and enjoy good health.

What Are The Best Foods For a Paleo Diet

Herbs, Spices, Extracts
High-antioxidant/ nutritional value
Sensible Indulgences
Dark chocolate, red wine
Supplements
Multi, omega-3, probiotics, vitamin d, protein/meal powder

Moderation Foods
Fruits - Locally grown, in-season, high-antioxidant (berries, pitted fruit)
High-Fat Dairy - Raw, fermented, unpasteurized
Starchy Tubers, Quinoa, Wild Rice - Athlete's carb option
Other Nuts, Seeds and Nut Butters - Great snack option

Healthy Fats
Animal fats, butter & coconut oil (cooking)
Avocados, coconut products, olives & olive oil, macadamias (eating)

Vegetables
Locally grown and/or organic. Abundant servings for flavor, nutrition, and antioxidants.

Meat • Fish • Fowl • Eggs
Bulk of dietary calories: saturated fat (energy, satiety, cell & hormone function) and protein (building blocks, lean mass). Emphasize local, pasture-raised or certified organic.

The paleo diet is based on a rough dietary plan modeled after what our ancestors may have consumed during the paleolithic era. The diet itself is extremely healthy and wholesome if adhered to. Thousands of people all over the world have reported many health benefits and positive results from adopting this diet. While the paleo diet may not be the panacea for all ills, it has numerous benefits.

The diet itself is pretty easy to understand conceptually. You have a list of foods that you can eat and a list of foods that you should not eat. It is very basic and anybody can understand it. Unlike other diets which use nutrient timings, food combinations, detoxes, lemonade, etc. the paleo diet is straightforward. However, it is not an easy diet to follow.
You'll need to be determined to get over the initial hump when your body is adjusting to the new foods. You will have cravings that will be gnawing at you constantly. Sugar cravings for the most part. Once you get past this, it will be smooth sailing.

So what are the best paleo foods?

The paleo foods you consume will be nutrient dense and natural. It is highly recommended that you eat organic produce and grass fed meats. Even eggs should be free range. However, this may prove to be expensive. So, if you cannot afford organic vegetables and grass fed meats, then by all means get the normal produce and meats. Most importantly, stick to the food list recommended by the diet.

There are many types of foods you can eat while on the paleo diet. It would be best to get a book on the paleo diet or paleo diet recipes to look at the options available to you. This article will give you a few suggestions, but it is by no means comprehensive. You will benefit more from research.

The following foods were recommended:
Meats – Poultry, Bacon, Pork, Ground Beef, Grass Fed Beef, Chicken Thigh, Chicken Leg, Chicken Wings, Turkey, Chicken Breast, Pork Tenderloin, Pork Chops, Steak, Veal, Lamb rack, Shrimp, Lobster, Clams, Salmon, Venison Steaks, Buffalo, New York Steak, Lamb Chops, Rabbit, Goat, Elk, Emu, Goose, Kangaroo, Bear, Beef Jerky, Eggs, Bison, Bison Steaks, Bison Jerky, Bison Ribeye, Bison Sirloin, Wild Boar, Reindeer, Turtle, Ostrich, Pheasant, Quail, Lean Veal, Chuck Steak, Rattlesnake

Now, of course you may balk at some of these foods and some might be next to impossible to obtain, but this is just a list. Pick and choose what you like and eat those. It does not have to be a rigid diet. Some flexibility is good.

Vegetables - Asparagus, Avocado, Artichoke hearts, Brussels sprouts, Carrots, Spinach, Celery, Broccoli, Zucchini, Cabbage, Peppers (All Kinds), Cauliflower, Parsley, Eggplant, Green Onions

Fats - Coconut oil, Olive oil, Macadamia Oil, Avocado Oil, Grass fed Butter

Nuts - Almonds, Cashews, Hazelnuts, Pecans, Pine Nuts, Pumpkin Seeds, Sunflower Seeds, Macadamia Nut, Walnuts
Fruit - Apple, Avocado, Blackberries, Papaya, Peaches, Plums, Mango, Lychee, Blueberries, Grapes, , Lemon, Strawberries, Watermelon, Pineapple, Guava, Lime, Raspberries, Cantaloupe, Tangerine, Figs, Oranges

If you consume only the foods on the list above, you will notice your health improve and you will look and feel better. Of course, always eat in moderation and not surfeit. If you eat sensibly and follow this diet, the results will be fantastic. Do give it a go.

Is the Paleo Lifestyle Sustainable?

Paleo Diet Menu Composition

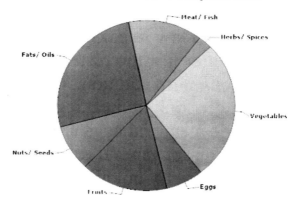

The paleo lifestyle often refers to adopting a paleo diet for life. This is often referred to as the 'cavemen' diet because it is how our early ancestors ate and lived. Several questions will come to people's minds when they first hear of the paleo diet. Is it healthy? Is it expensive? Why do I have to sacrifice my favorite foods? Is it uncivilized?

All these questions are often based on misconceptions and false notions. The paleo diet though slightly restrictive is perfectly healthy and sustainable. As with anything that needs to become a habit, it will take some time to adapt to the paleo diet and make it a way of life.

Most diets are not sustainable in the long run. They are either too low in calories, based on false information or just too restrictive and not feasible for a long term solution. The paleo diet recommends a diet rich in meat, eggs and healthy fats. The meat and eggs are best if they are organic. Grains, sugar and refined or processed foods are strictly not allowed. This is where most people face the biggest hurdle.

Giving up their favorite foods such as chocolates, cakes, pastries, ice-creams, etc. is such a sacrifice. Is it even worth it? This is a question every individual will need to answer for themselves. There are paleo recipes to make desserts, smoothies and even ice-creams. So, it's not that bad but of course, you'll have to forget the Dunkin Donuts.

You'll have to decide if you want good health and a lean, fit body. The good thing about the paleo diet is that after you have been on it for 3 months, your cravings for sweet foods will diminish greatly. A lot of your past cravings will not be there anymore. You will not feel the need to raid the refrigerator at night and binge eat. When the body has all the nutrients it needs, it doesn't have sudden cravings. So, in the long run, it will not seem like a sacrifice at all.

The paleo diet is not more expensive than a normal diet. You are just substituting foods. In fact, since the paleo diet often recommends that you buy your meats and fresh foods in bulk, often there will be cost savings. You are also encouraged to cook for yourself.

That means overall, you will be saving money. Any savvy paleo dieter will be able to adroitly get better bargains from his local meat suppliers. The only investment you will have to make is on a freezer to store your meats. This, however, is a one-time investment that will last for years.

So, to summarize, the paleo diet is actually cheaper than the standard American diet. Not to mention, you will save on medical costs since you will be less susceptible to the normal health issues that affect most people on a poor diet.

The paleo diet is definitely sustainable in the long run. You will benefit from it greatly. The only difficulty is in the beginning when you are first getting used to it. Once you cross the hump, it will be smooth sailing the rest of the way and you'll realize that the paleo lifestyle is an excellent way to live.

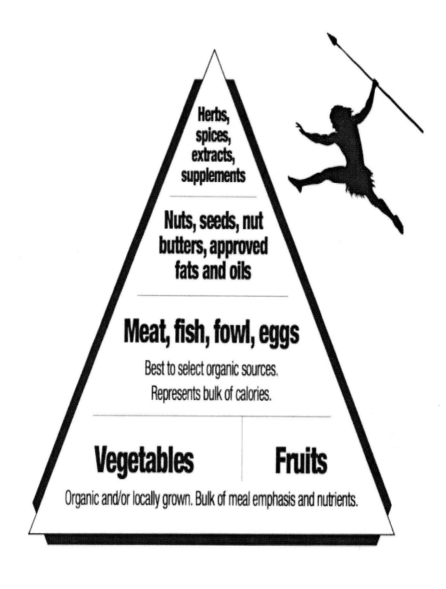

Herbs, spices, extracts, supplements

Nuts, seeds, nut butters, approved fats and oils

Meat, fish, fowl, eggs

Best to select organic sources.
Represents bulk of calories.

Vegetables | Fruits

Organic and/or locally grown. Bulk of meal emphasis and nutrients.

The Ultimate Paleo Guide

Recommends that you visit:

www.eatinghealthytoloseweight.net

Is It More Expensive To Go On a Paleo Diet?

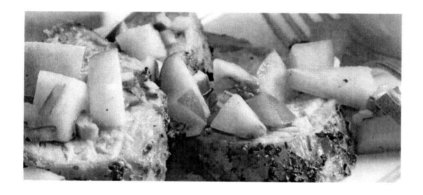

The paleo diet is often to be more costly than just being on a normal diet. In fact, this is one of the reasons many people do not get on it. However, the paleo diet does not necessarily have to be expensive. You just need to tailor it to your needs. One of the requirements of the paleo diet is to consume organic foods and grass-fed meats. There is absolutely no doubt that these are more expensive than normal meats. So what do you do?

Simple. You just adapt the paleo diet to suit your lifestyle and budget. There is absolutely no need to be so strict. The rules are not written in stone. Have some flexibility. You cannot afford free range eggs? No problem. Just eat normal eggs. You can't afford grass-fed beef? Then get the normal lean cuts of beef.

These options are better than just sacrificing the eggs and getting a box of doughnuts instead. Your food choices are what really matters. That is the crux of the diet. Consuming what is on the list only and not the foods that aren't allowed. You may easily switch to organic foods when you have the money. Choosing to buy grass fed beef when you have money is way easier than giving up a life of eating junk food.

You are advised to get a large freezer to store your meats which you would be buying in bulk. No money for a freezer? No problem. Slowly save up for one. This is a one-time investment and will last you for years. You are also advised to buy your meats and groceries in bulk. This usually will result in cost savings if you do your due diligence and look for the best prices.

It is often assumed that since you are buying in bulk, you'll spend more. This is true. However, the food will last for at least 2 weeks. So, you might only be doing grocery shopping twice a month. The difficulty arises from having enough money to spend on 2 weeks worth of grocery shopping at one go since it is a sizeable chunk of change. Yet, this is mostly an illusion.

At the end of the month you will be spending roughly the same amount if you do your shopping every 3 days or twice a month. In fact, you'll be spending less shopping just twice a month. So, save up till you can afford to spend on grocery shopping at one go for 2 weeks. The chances of you actually seeing cost savings are highly propitious.

The paleo diet is not more expensive. It takes some adjusting to but that is only in the initial phase. Once you have money for a freezer and enough for bulk purchases, you will find that the diet is actually cheaper. Make the diet suit you and not the other way around. Adhere to the important fundamentals such as proper food choices. The frills can wait till you have cash to do so. Do not give up on this diet. It is awesome.

ONE WEEK MEAL PLAN

Day	Breakfast	Lunch	Dinner	Side Dish	Snack	Dessert
Mon	Buffalo Strip Steak with Veggies and Bacon	Mango Chicken Salad with Chipotle Mayo	Seriously Tasty Paleo Meat Loaf	Smashed Plantains	Pecan Pie Butter with Apples	Chocolate Zucchini Brownies
Tue	Stir Fried Kale and Bacon	Seriously Tasty Paleo Meat Loaf	Slow Cooker Chicken	Chipotle Slaw	Smoked Salmon Nori Roll	Apple Muffins
Wed	Breakfast Squash and Sausage	Laksa Lemak	Melt in Your Mouth Beef Stew	Jicama Salad with Cilantro Lime Vinaigrette	Tuna Stuffed Avocado	Berries and Coconut Whipped Cream
Thu	Jicama and Sausage Breakfast Pie	Basque Lamb Stew	Beef Stew	Carrot and Parsnip Puree	Crunchy Crackers	Almond Butter Bliss with Cacao Nibs
Fri	Bratwurst and German	Jambalaya	Garlic Chicken with White Wine Sauce	Cauliflower Stuffed Acorn Squash	Taro Chips	Cacao Brownies
Sat	Rutabaga and Onion Sat Hash Browns	Grilled or Broiled Filet Mignon with Red Wine Sauce	Moroccan Chicken Salad	Celeriac and Rutabaga Puree	Jerky	Banana-cado Chocolate Pudding
Sun	Seared Fish with Beets and Broccoli	Slow Cooker Pork Pot Roast	Baked Tilapia with Lemon and Thyme	Cucumber Wakame Salad	Jerky	Coconut Pineapple Upside

9 / 20

The Ultimate Paleo Guide

Recommends that you visit:

www.eatinghealthytoloseweight.net

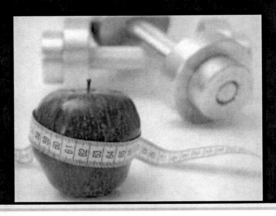

Controlling Cravings While On the Paleo Diet

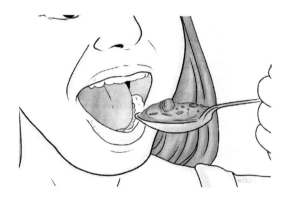

Controlling Cravings While On the Paleo Diet

The paleo diet is considered one of the healthiest diets on the planets. It is extremely popular among fitness fanatics who swear by its effectiveness. Unlike most other fad diets on the market, the paleo diet does not overly concern itself with calories or detoxing or even macronutrients.

The paleo diet is more about making the correct food choices. Grains, processed foods, sugar and a few other foods are not allowed in the paleo diet. This is a slightly restrictive diet. Not overly so. However, the foods that are not allowed are often very close to people's hearts. The elimination of sugar means that comfort foods such as ice-creams, cakes, chocolates, etc. are not allowed. Most people cannot even imagine life without indulging in these foods. Junk food is also not allowed.

It is this issue that has made so many people fall off the paleo bandwagon. They started off with good intentions but gave up when their cravings got the better of them. This article will show you a few ways to control your cravings. The methods below will help a great deal but you need to be aware, that the cravings will still be there. The best consolation is that with time, these cravings will disappear. Your body is just used to years of poor food choices and it will take some time to change the way you eat. The best habits take time to be inculcated. Rest assured that if you stay the course, you will control your cravings and one day, they will be a thing of your past.

The best way to control cravings for sweet foods will be to have some sweet foods on standby. Really? Yes… But, these will be paleo sweet foods. There are several paleo recipes for smoothies, ice-creams and other desserts that you can find in a paleo cookbook. You may be surprised but a strong craving for chocolate may be diminished by eating a cold, slice of watermelon. You'll just need to find paleo substitutes for sweet foods. Keep a few on standby at all times. You never know when you may get a craving. When it hits you, just consume the substitute.

Another way to control cravings will be to remove all the food in your house that does not fit in with your paleo diet. Don't create temptation. Having a big tub of chocolate ice-cream in the freezer is just asking for trouble. Get rid of all these potential problems. Don't test your will power.

Bring your own cooked food to work. In the beginning, when you're first starting a paleo diet, it will be good to avoid eating with friends. Looking at their food is going to give you cravings, unless they are also on a paleo diet. Often, people eat at restaurants or diners together and these are best avoided. It may seem anti-social in the beginning, but it's only for about 2 or 3 months till you have conquered your cravings.

The paleo diet is not easy to adopt. It has a very steep learning curve. So, you need to be aware of the initial problems. However, once you have gotten used to it, you will wish you had started on it sooner. The best things in life require effort and the paleo diet is one of them.

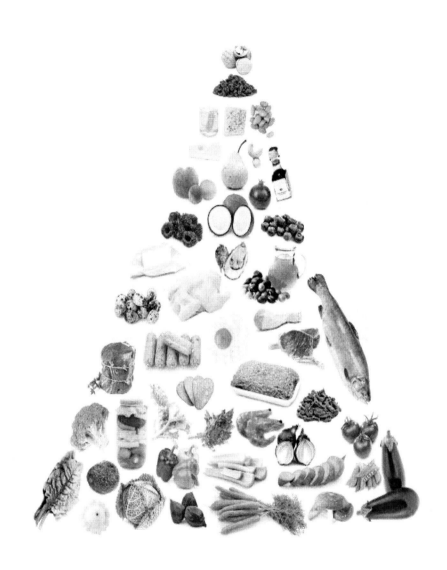

The Ultimate Paleo Guide

Recommends that you visit:

www.eatinghealthytoloseweight.net

7 Benefits of Adopting the Paleo Diet

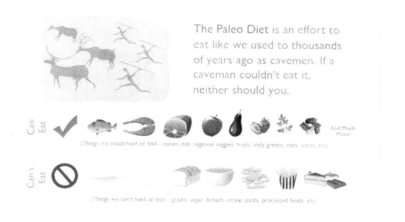

The Paleo Diet is an effort to eat like we used to thousands of years ago as cavemen. If a caveman couldn't eat it, neither should you.

Can Eat ✓ (Things we could hunt or find – meats, fish, regional veggies, fruits, leafy greens, nuts, seeds, etc)   And Much More!

Can't Eat 🚫 (Things we can't hunt or find – grains, sugar, breads, cereal, pasta, processed foods, etc.)

There are many benefits to adopting the paleo diet. This article will state seven but this list is by no means exhaustive. There are many more positive effects and gains to be achieved from switching to the paleo diet.

The paleo diet can quite simply be defined as a very wholesome diet which only allows the consumption of natural foods such as meat, vegetables and healthy fats such as coconut oils, macadamia oils, olive oils, etc. It forbids the consumption of grains, grain based food products, sugar and any kind of processed food.

Natural all the way. That is the key to the paleo diet. Of course, taste need not be sacrificed. Spices may be used and there are several excellent paleo recipe books on the market which will teach you to whip up healthy yet tasty dishes.

The first benefit to the paleo diet will be a reduced risk of disease. The current diet most people are used to is loaded with preservatives, harmful additives and other artificial ingredients that cause all kinds of health problems and obesity. Switching to the paleo diet will eliminate most of these problems.

The second benefit will be a loss of excess fat. The paleo diet aims to reduce the amount of carbohydrates you consume. This will keep your blood sugar levels stable and increase your insulin sensitivity. That means your body will be more responsive to burning off fat and staying lean.

The reduction of inflammation is the third benefit. Thousands of people all over the world complain of daily aches and pains. Their body hurts but they do not know why. The reason is inflammation due to the consumption of unhealthy foods. The cells are inflamed from the food they ate. By switching to the paleo diet, you will be consuming a very healthy diet. This will reduce all inflammation and increase your sense of well-being.

The fourth benefit is increased muscle mass. Since the paleo diet revolves around the consumption of copious amounts of meat, you will be getting a lot of protein. This will aid in muscle growth and recovery, if you engage in regular exercise. There will be much less muscle breakdown. The more muscle you have, the more calories you burn. This basically means that you will be lean, fit and healthy.

A healthier brain and organs are the fifth benefit. Our body needs omega-3 fatty acids to be healthy. However, the modern diet today has seen an overload of omega-6 fatty acids and a drastic reduction in the healthier omega-3 acids. By consuming healthy meats such as grass-fed meats, eggs and wild caught salmon, you will be giving your body a healthy dose of omega-3 acids.

The sixth benefit is reduced tendency to get allergies. Modern day foods contain ingredients that raise people's sensitivity to allergens. By cutting out these foods, our ability to get allergies is greatly reduced.

The seventh benefit is increased energy. Initially, the diet may be a little difficult to follow and you will not feel so good because your body is ridding itself of toxins accumulated from past eating habits. The change in diet also can be challenging. However, once you get over this hump, it will be smooth sailing all the way. You will find yourself full of life and bursting with energy.

The above seven reasons should be good enough to persuade you to give the paleo diet a try. You may never look back and most people on the paleo diet say that it is one of the best things they ever did.

Ways to Boost Your Health While On the Paleo Diet

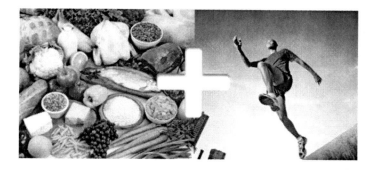

The paleo diet is one of the most popular diets around. Unlike most other diets which are just fads, unsustainable in the long run or ineffective, the paleo diet is highly effective and a long term solution to a leaner and healthier body.

The paleo diet is low on sodium and sugar but high in protein and moderate with the carb intake. This is exactly why it is so effective in weight loss and keeping other health issues in check.

Obesity is a growing problem in the US and around the world. The paleo diet, if strictly followed, will definitely ameliorate this problem. Nothing but good can come from giving up processed and refined foods in favor of wholesome, healthy, natural foods. Your blood sugar levels will be stable and you will be much healthier.

Of course, the paleo diet is not a be all and end all to good health. There are a few other factors to consider that will ensure all round good health when combined with the paleo diet.

1. Sufficient sleep

   All too often people sacrifice precious sleep to squeeze in more living into their day. The problem is, in most cases, sleep is sacrificed for the television, surfing the internet, late night partying, etc.

   Over time, this will take a toll on one's health. Burning the candle at both ends is never a good idea and sooner or later, your body will suffer the ill effects of sleep deprivation. Always ensure that you get enough sleep.

2. Engage in resistance training

Men and women alike will benefit from resistance training. Stronger muscles are always a good thing. Weight training has multiple benefits from stronger ligaments, increased metabolism and even slows down the aging process. It is not a man's thing. Women too should train with weights.

3. Do at least 3 sessions of cardio a week

Cardio activity is crucial to good health. Your cardiovascular system requires constant training. Any activity that raises your heart rate for 20 minutes continuously can be considered a cardio activity. Find one that you like and do it thrice a week for about 20 to 30 minutes. It could be walking, running, cycling, rowing, skipping, anything that you like.

4. Cook for yourself

It is understandable that cooking can be a hassle in today's fast paced world. There just does not seem to be enough time. It is highly recommended that you cook in large amounts. For example, you could cook on Sunday for the whole week or just for the next 3 days. It's up to you. If you cook for yourself, you will know exactly what goes into your food and if it's nutritious. You'll also save money in the long run.

5. Learn more paleo recipes

The paleo diet, though slightly restrictive, does not have to be bland. There are many excellent cookbooks on the market dedicated to paleo recipes. Grab a book and try out the recipes. Your food will taste better and you'll have variety. This will go a long way in making sure you stick with the paleo diet.

These are just a few methods you can use to improve your health and see faster results while on the paleo diet. You will lose weight faster, look better and feel great if you use the above tips while on the paleo diet.

5 Paleo Diet Tips You Must Know

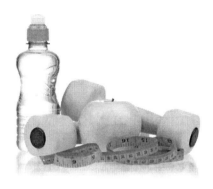

The paleo diet has become one of the latest fitness 'crazes' around. Those who have adopted it swear by its effectiveness and extol its life changing benefits. Others however, feel like it is better suited for feral cavemen.
So what is the paleo diet?

The paleo diet, also known as the caveman diet, is a nutritional plan similar to what our early ancestors who lived during the Paleolithic era followed. Basically, the consumption of natural foods such as fish, grass-fed pasture raised meats, fruit, fungi, eggs, vegetables, roots, and nuts. The diet excludes grains, legumes, dairy products, potatoes, refined salt, refined sugar, and processed oils.

Is it effective?

Definitely. It is an extremely healthy diet and the health benefits are many.
This article will highlight 5 paleo diet tips you should be aware of to help you get the best out of this fantastic way of life.

1. Use spices effectively and wisely.
   Since the paleo diet does not allow for sauces and other refined products, you will need to learn how to use spices effectively to season your food. One of the major causes for people giving up the paleo diet is due to the fact that the food tastes bland.

   This is true if you do not use spices to flavor your food. The East Indians are very good at using spices to prepare their dishes. The food is aromatic, tasty and the spices have various medicinal properties too. So, learn how to flavor your food using spices.

2. Vary Your Veggies

Consume a wide variety of vegetables. It is common to just stick with one vegetable and go by a week eating only that. Since most people who adopt the paleo diet buy their food in bulk, it's so much easier to just dump four large broccolis in the cart and walk to checkout. If you do that, you'll be missing out the benefits that other veggies will bring you.

Consume different vegetables of different colors. Kale, spinach, cabbage, eggplant, carrots, etc. are all excellent choices. Do try them.

3. Pre-cook Your Food

The best way to stay focused on your paleo diet will be to pre-cook your food in batches and keep them in the refrigerator. It is advisable to cook for 3 or 4 days in advance. Preparing paleo meals is fast and easy. So, you can do this once or twice a week.

When your food is all prepared and ready, it is much easier to just take a pre-prepared meal to work. The idea of cooking daily is can be quite demoralizing. Being unprepared or if you're suddenly short on time will lead to difficult decisions and you may even have to eat food you're not supposed to.

4. Don't Create Temptation

   Do not keep junk food such as ice-cream, cakes, chocolates, etc. in your house. You will be tempted and that makes things much harder.

5. Learn To Make Paleo Smoothies and Other Treats

   The paleo diet is not a boring one. It is slightly restrictive but there are many recipes available online that will teach you how to make smoothies and even ice-cream to satisfy your sweet tooth.

   Learn more and try more recipes out. Knowledge is power and with the knowledge, you will be able to make your paleo lifestyle fun, sustainable and rewarding in the long run.

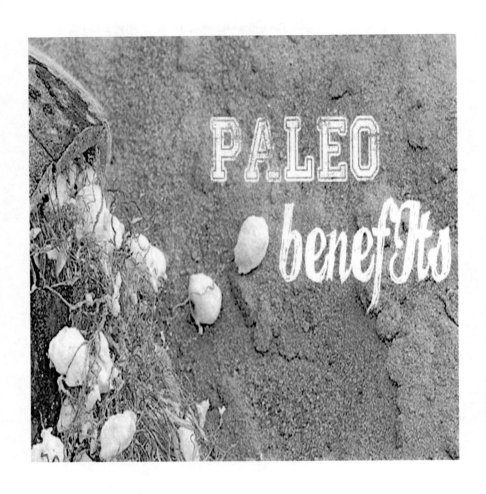

5 Common Misconceptions about the Paleo Diet

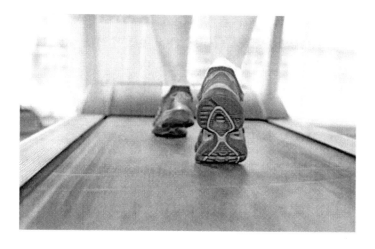

Even though the paleo diet has thousands of followers, seen a surge in popularity and has been around for a few years, there are many misconceptions about this diet. These misconceptions arise through false information, a bad image of paleo dieting and even marketing attempts by other fad diets to discredit the paleo way.

The paleo diet is also known as the 'caveman' diet. This is due to the fact that the diet somewhat resembles the way our early ancestors ate. This name has caused one of the biggest misconceptions about the paleo diet.

1. It is uncivilized and all about gorging yourself on meat

   The paleo diet is about eating nutrient rich food that does not contain harmful substances and agrees with our body. It is not a re-enactment of how the actual cavemen ate. Paleo dieters do not go out hunting for boars or deer and roast the meat on a flame.

   The diet is about eating the correct foods and excluding the bad ones. Grains, sugar, processed foods, etc. are not allowed. This is due to the fact that these foods are neither natural nor healthy. There are millions of people who have problems with grain based foods. So, the diet is not only about meat. Vegetables, healthy fats and fruit may be consumed too.

2. Paleo dieting is for fat loss

Fat loss is one of the benefits of a paleo diet but it is not the goal. Unlike the Atkins diet or other low carb diets, the paleo diet is not overly concerned about weight loss. The concept of the paleo diet is to consume wholesome, healthy food and stop eating detrimental food.

Once this is achieved, weight loss naturally follows. Obesity is a growing trend around the world and it is reaching epidemic proportions. That's because of poor food choices. The paleo diet is a healthy way to eat and live. It is more than just fat loss.

3. The paleo diet is not practical
   The paleo diet does require some effort and preparation. That does not make it impractical. You just need to find ways to make it easier for you. Cooking your food for a few days at a time, pre-packing them in containers for ease, etc. If you are truly dedicated, you will find a way.

4. The paleo diet is expensive

No, it's not. You are encouraged to buy your meat and vegetables from farmers' markets and other suppliers. Usually, you may receive discounts and other special rates. Since you will be doing your own cooking, you'll be spending less on food. Furthermore, since you can't consume junk food and processed food, you will not be spending on the usual comforts foods. So, the paleo diet could actually be cheaper.

5. The paleo diet is not for women
   There are many arguments for this stating that women need more carbohydrates, etc. In cases like this, it would be wise to adapt the diet. For example, if the woman feels lethargic, she may consume more carbs in the form of vegetables. The paleo diet does not have to be rigid. Mix and match and see what suits you.

These are just a few misconceptions. There are many more but pay them no heed. The best way to know about anything is to try it out for yourself. Try out the paleo diet for 3 weeks or a month. If you start looking and feeling better, stay on. If not, you may go back to your previous way of eating. Chances are high that once you go paleo, you'll never go back.

The Real Skinny about the Paleo Diet

The Paleo Diet is all about NATURAL foods to help achieve great health and a perfect physique!

The human body evolved for more than 2 million years with food found in nature...

game meats | fish | vegetables | wild fruit | eggs | nuts

The paleo diet has its fair share of fans and detractors. The diet itself has gained massive popularity over the years and thousands of people swear by it. They often claim to feel much better and healthier as a result of adopting this diet. Thousands of people have also lost weight by adopting the paleo diet, which is also known as the 'caveman' diet.

The diet basically focuses on eating single ingredient foods such as fish, grass fed meat, goat, poultry, rabbit and a lot of other meats. You are also encouraged to consume a variety of vegetables from broccolis, carrots, cabbages, etc. Contrary to popular diets, the paleo diet also encourages the consumption of healthy fats such as coconut oil, olive oil, macadamia oil, grass fed butter, etc. The emphasis is on wholesome, nutritious foods that our early ancestors ate during the paleolithic era.

Grains, refined and processed foods, sugar and other modern foods that the typical American consumes is anathema to the avid paleo dieter. They are not allowed to consume these foods at all as part of the paleo diet.

The trend in obesity has skyrocketed and it has reached epidemic proportions. Thousands and thousands of Americans are obese and the food industry is to blame. Paleo dieters have dumped the Standard American Diet, which is known as SAD amongst paleo fans, for a healthier alternative.

The results prove that the paleo diet works. Thousands of testimonials show that people have lost weight using this method. They report feeling much better ever since they stopped eating grains and process foods such as white bread or products which are marketed as 'healthy' by billion dollar food manufacturers.

Going natural has made a world of difference to the paleo dieters.

Now, of course there are people who say that the paleo diet is not healthy because you will not get all the nutrients your body needs. This is not true. The only time that your body lacks nutrients is if you do not consume a varied diet. By eating a variety of foods, your body will have all the nutrients it needs.

Another point that detractors may throw up is that consuming too much meat and eggs will raise your cholesterol level. However, studies have shown that dietary cholesterol has minimal impact on your blood cholesterol level. The real culprit is modern day foods that inflame the body and cause cholesterol to be formed to heal the inflamed cells.

On another tangent, there are folks who say that the paleo diet is uncivilized. This is purely an image issue. The fact that the diet is modeled after a caveman's diet and is actually called that, conjures up images of feral men tearing into raw meat in some caves.

This is just a psychological issue. Most paleo dieters just eat more meat and they cook it well, spice it up and in many cases, their food tastes just as good as or even better than a greasy steak you may find at a local diner.

The crux of the matter is that the paleo diet is extremely beneficial to one's health. The saying, 'Don't knock it till you try it' applies here. It will do you good to give it a try and you just might find yourself a fan of this remarkable diet.

The Ultimate Paleo Guide

Recommends that you visit:

www.eatinghealthytoloseweight.net

CPSIA information can be obtained at www.ICGtesting.com
Printed in the USA
BVOW03s1122260415

397742BV00019B/461/P